MY ultimate RECIPES

foreword

Cooking makes you HAPPY. YES! Because you create something by yourself. With your own hands. Something to be proud of. Good food is a joy. Himself. Or his loved one. Cooking is always a small event, a small highlight in the evening that you look forward to. Where you can switch off and truly enjoy the End of the day. That's why cooking makes you HAPPY. And because happy people make our planet a better place, there are delicious recipes. This is our small humble notebook for your tasty food.

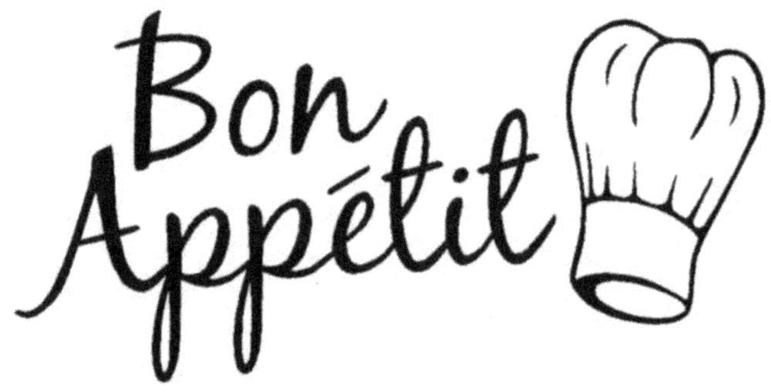

small Recipes

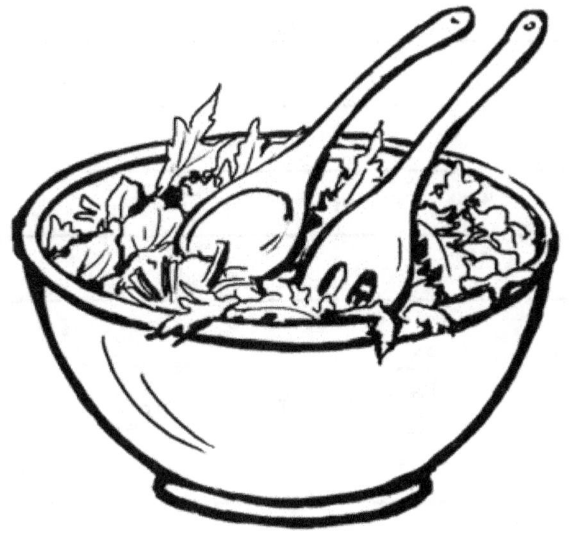

1. Recipe

Ingredients:

Method:

2. Recipe

Real

Ingredients:

____

____

____

____

____

Method:

____

____

____

____

____

____

3. Recipe

Ingredients:

Method:

4. Recipe

Ingredients:

____

____

____

____

____

Method:

____

____

____

____

____

____

____

5. Recipe

Ingredients:

Method:

6. Recipe

Ingredients:

Method:

7. Recipe

Ingredients:

Method:

8. Recipe

Ingredients:

Method:

9. Recipe

Ingredients:

Method:

10. Recipe

Ingredients:

____

____

____

____

____

____

Method:

____

____

____

____

____

____

____

____

11. Recipe

Ingredients:

Method:

12.   Recipe

Ingredients:

Method:

13.   Recipe

Ingredients:

Method:

14.   Recipe

Ingredients:

____

____

____

____

____

Method:

____

____

____

____

____

____

15. Recipe

Ingredients:

Method:

16.   Recipe

Ingredients:

Method:

17.   Recipe

Ingredients:

Method:

18.   Recipe

Ingredients:

____

____

____

____

____

Method:

____

____

____

____

____

____

____

19.   Recipe

Ingredients:

____

____

____

____

____

____

Method:

____

____

____

____

____

____

____

20.   Recipe

Ingredients:

____

____

____

____

____

____

Method:

____

____

____

____

____

____

____

21.   Recipe

Ingredients:

Method:

22.   Recipe

Ingredients:

Method:

23.   Recipe

Ingredients:

____

____

____

____

____

____

Method:

____

____

____

____

____

____

____

24.   Recipe

Kcal

Ingredients:

____

____

____

____

____

____

Method:

____

____

____

____

____

____

____

25.   Recipe

Kcal ....

Ingredients:

____
____
____
____
____

Method: ....

____
____
____
____
____
____

26.   Recipe

Ingredients:

Method:

27.   Recipe

Kcal

Ingredients:

____

____

____

____

____

Method:

____

____

____

____

____

____

28.   Recipe

Ingredients:

Method:

29.   Recipe

Kcal

Ingredients:

Method:

30.   Recipe

Ingredients:

____

____

____

____

____

____

Method:

____

____

____

____

____

____

____

____

31.   Recipe

Ingredients:

____

____

____

____

____

____

Method:

____

____

____

____

____

____

____

32.   Recipe

Ingredients:

____

____

____

____

____

Method:

____

____

____

____

____

____

33.   Recipe

Ingredients:

____

Method:

34. Recipe

Ingredients:

Method:

35.   Recipe

Ingredients:

____

____

____

____

____

____

Method:

____

____

____

____

____

____

____

36.   Recipe

Ingredients:

Method:

37.   Recipe

Ingredients:

Method:

38.   Recipe

Ingredients:

Method:

39.   Recipe

Ingredients:

Method:

40.   Recipe

Ingredients:

Method:

41.   Recipe

Ingredients:

Method:

42.   Recipe

Ingredients:

____

____

____

____

____

Method:

____

____

____

____

____

____

____

43.   Recipe

Ingredients:

Method:

44.   Recipe

Ingredients:

____

____

____

____

____

____

Method:

____

____

____

____

____

____

____

45. Recipe

Ingredients:

____
____
____
____
____
____

Method:

____
____
____
____
____
____
____

46.　　Recipe

Ingredients:

____

____

____

____

____

Method:

____

____

____

____

____

____

____

47.   Recipe

Ingredients:

____

____

____

____

____

____

Method:

____

____

____

____

____

____

____

48.   Recipe

Ingredients:

____

____

____

____

____

Method:

____

____

____

____

____

____

49.   Recipe

Kcal

Ingredients:

Method:

50.   Recipe

Ingredients:

Method:

51.   Recipe

Kcal

Ingredients:

Method:

52.   Recipe

Kcal

Ingredients:

Method:

53.   Recipe

Kcal

Ingredients:

____

____

____

____

____

____

Method:

____

____

____

____

____

____

____

____

54.   Recipe

Kcal

![spoon and fork notebook] **Ingredients:**

____

____

____

____

____

____

Method:

____

____

____

____

____

____

____

55.   Recipe

Ingredients:

Method:

Big Reripes

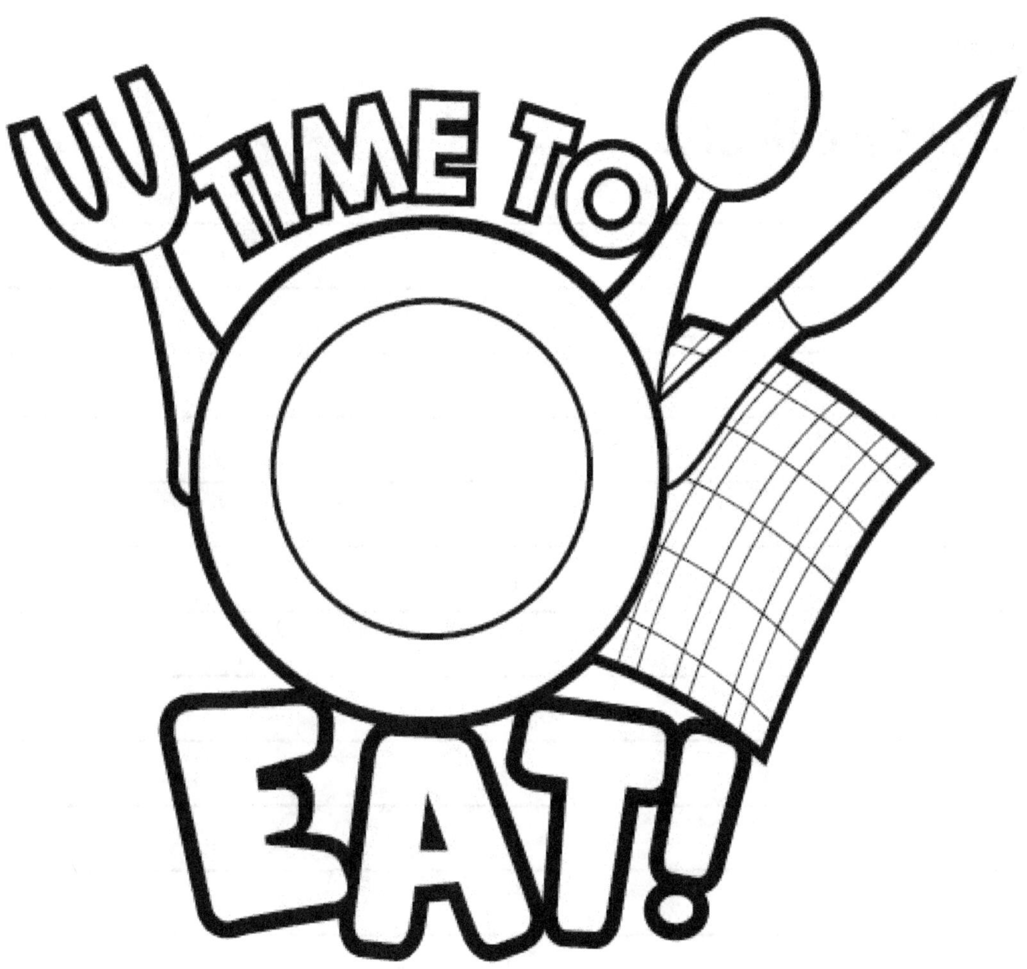

56.   Recipe

Kcal

Ingredients:

➡️

Method:

Recipe Tips

57.   Recipe

Kcal

Ingredients:

Method:

Recipe Tips

58.   Recipe

Kcal

Ingredients:

Method:

Recipe Tips

59.   Recipe

Kcal

Ingredients:

Method:

Recipe Tips

60.   Recipe

Kcal

Ingredients:

Method:

Recipe Tips

61.   Recipe

Ingredients:

Method:

Recipe Tips

62.   Recipe

Kcal

Ingredients:

Method:

Recipe Tips

63.   Recipe

Kcal

Ingredients:

____

Method:

Recipe Tips

64.   Recipe

Ingredients:

Kcal

Method:

Recipe Tips

65.   Recipe

Ingredients:

Method:

Recipe Tips

66.   Recipe

Kcal

Ingredients:

____

____

____

____

____

____

____

____

____

____

____

Method:

Recipe Tips

67.   Recipe

Kcal

Ingredients:

Method:

Recipe Tips

68.   Recipe

Kcal

Ingredients:

Method:

Recipe Tips

69.   Recipe

Ingredients:

Method:

Recipe Tips

70.   Recipe

Ingredients:

Method:

Recipe Tips

71.   Recipe

Ingredients:

____

____

____

____

____

____

____

____

____

____

Method:

Recipe Tips

72.　Recipe

Ingredients:

Method:

Recipe Tips

Ingredients:

____

____

____

____

____

____

____

____

____

____

Method:

Recipe Tips

74.   Recipe

Ingredients:

Method:

75.   Recipe

Ingredients:

____

____

____

____

____

____

____

____

____

____

Method:

Recipe Tips

76.   Recipe

Kcal

Ingredients:

____

____

____

____

____

____

____

____

____

____

Method:

Recipe Tips

77. Recipe

Kcal

Ingredients:

Method:

Recipe Tips

78. Recipe

Kcal

Ingredients:

Method:

Recipe Tips

Kcal

Ingredients:

Method:

Recipe Tips

80.   Recipe

Ingredients:

Method:

Recipe Tips

81.　　Recipe

Ingredients:

Method:

____

Recipe Tips

82.   Recipe

Ingredients:

Method:

Recipe Tips

83.   Recipe

Kcal

Ingredients:

Method: ....

Recipe Tips

84.   Recipe

Ingredients:

Method:

Recipe Tips

85. Recipe

Kcal

Ingredients:

____
____
____
____
____
____
____
____
____
____

Method:

Recipe Tips

Notes:

Symbolverzeichnis

 ready in

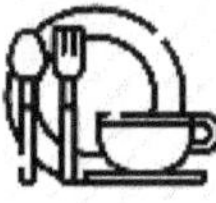 numbre of serves

 Calories per serving

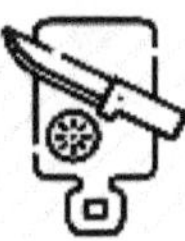 prepation time

 cooking time

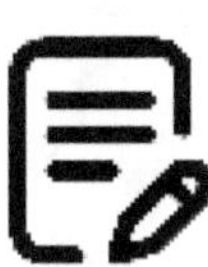 Notes

www.ingramcontent.com/pod-product-compliance
Lightning Source LLC
Chambersburg PA
CBHW081437250726
48662CB00009B/2829